Fast and Easy Acid Reflux Diet and Remedies

"Get a life without pain and discomfort with these reflux remedies."

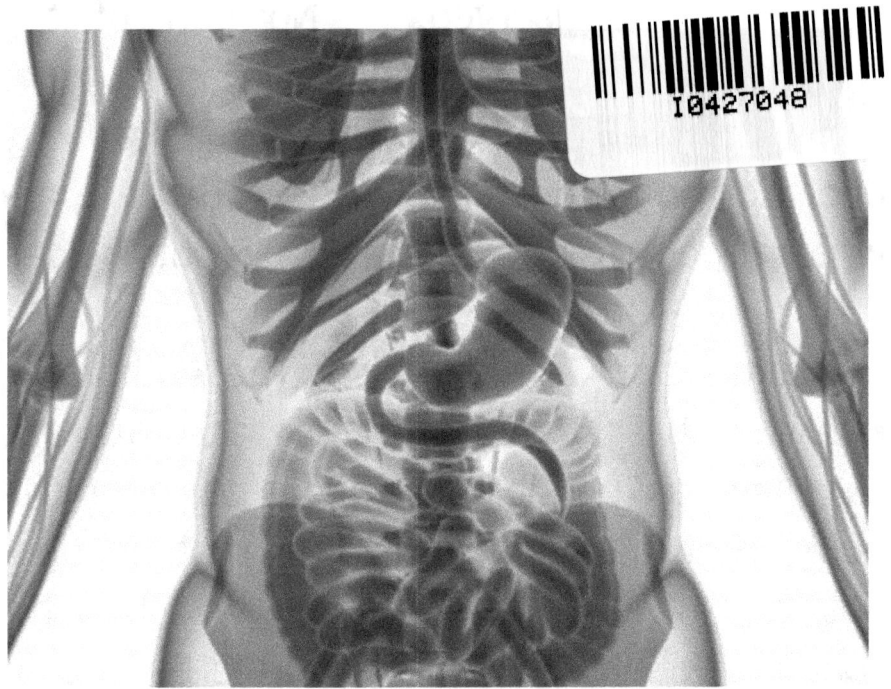

Rudy S. Silva, Natural Nutritionist

Fastest and Easiest Cures for Acid Reflux ©
First printing 2011, Second Printing 2013,
Third Printing 2018, by Rudy S. Silva,

ISBN-13:978-1492920212
ISBN-10: 1492920215

Disclaimer and Terms of Use: The Author and Publisher has strived to be as accurate and complete as possible in the creation of this book, notwithstanding the fact that he does not warrant or represent at any time that the contents within are accurate due to the rapidly changing nature of the Internet. While all attempts have been made to verify information provided in this publication, the Author and Publisher assumes no responsibility for errors, omissions, or contrary interpretation of the subject matter herein. Any perceived slights of specific persons, peoples, or organizations are unintentional.

Your doctor or health provider should confirm any information given here. This information should not be taken as medical advice or treatment. This e-book is for information and educational purposes only.

Printed in the United States of America, 2011, 2013, 2018.

Table of Contents

1: Acid Reflux Explained

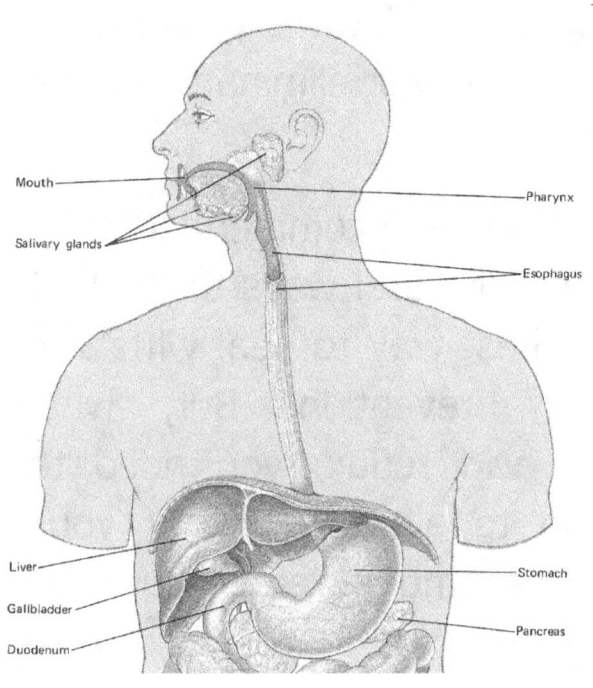

Acid Reflux and GERD

Most people know what heartburn or indigestion feels like or when they have acid reflux. But, there may be some confusion about what acid reflux and GERD, gastro esophageal reflux disease, really is. In this ebook, you will discover the difference between these acid reflux conditions. And, you will discover what causes acid reflux, what the symptoms are, and what you need to do to reduce, overcome, or eliminate acid reflux.

Most of what is recommended in this book is how to use natural ways to deal with acid reflux. The best way to deal with acid reflux is through prevention. But, when you experience acid reflux, you need to know what to do to alleviate it. If your reflux symptoms become severe, you should see your doctor.

It is a good idea to see your doctor when you are dealing with continual acid reflux in this way you can become aware of how severe your condition is. When you know this, then you will know what natural remedies you need to use in conjunction with what your doctor recommends.

So What Is Acid Reflux?

Acid reflux is a condition where some of your stomach content flows back up into your esophagus. There is a "muscle valve" at the top of your stomach that typical prevents stomach content from flowing back into your esophagus. However, when this muscle valve, 3 to 4 cm area, called Lower Esophagus Sphincter, LES, becomes weak, it can't hold back your stomach content.

In addition, a weak valve with excess stomach gas pressure is a definite condition for acid reflux. But, a high stomach gas pressure can, also, open a strong LES and allow stomach content to push back into your esophagus and throat. This kind of strong backward flow occurs when you vomit from eating contaminated food.

Acid reflux occurs when your stomach rejects the mixture of food you have eaten or is unable to properly digest it. Excess gases form in your stomach from undigested food, forcing your LES to open. The gas pressure forces food into your esophagus cause a burning sensation.

The burning occurs from the stomach acid attacking your esophagus lining. This burning sensation can be felt from the top of your throat down to near the bottom of your rib cage.

There are cases where no burning sensation occurs when stomach content move into your esophagus. In this case there are certain symptoms that occur with this condition. This type of acid reflux is referred to as "Silent Acid Reflux." This condition will be addressed in the coming chapters.

Silent Acid Reflux

Silent acid reflux occurs when stomach contents, which is acidic, flows into the esophagus and starts to burn the sensitive tissue there. The burning is felt below the collar bone. Sometimes this burning or pain can be mistaken for heart pain.

There are millions of Americans that have silent acid reflux without don't know it, and even their doctors misdiagnose it. They may have the reflux symptoms, but their symptoms are mistaken for other conditions.

So what is GERD?

Gastro esophageal reflux disease or GERD is a severe case of acid reflux, which results from a poor lifestyle. If you have acid reflux regularly, one to two times a week, then you have GERD.

If you have acid reflux, heartburn or what they call GERD, you probably have been abusing your stomach, and body, by eating poorly, taking medication, using excess pain killers, not sleeping eight hours, or not exercising much.

If you have been experiencing acid reflux weekly consider this a serious issue, since this condition can turn into a detrimental disease.

Using Drugs for Acid Reflux

"Recently I got an email from a woman who said her male friend was taken to the emergency and was found to have bleeding in the esophagus lining. This was a result of advanced heartburn. (GERD)

Apparently, he also had been taking Aleve for a year or so, and the doctors found he had severe liver damage. He typically drank 2-3 beers a day, so the combination of unhealthy living finally caught up with him, and now his liver may be irreparable."

You may think that this just couldn't happen to you. You don't do live like this. But, if you look around you, most people as they age are coming down with a variety of deadly diseases that eventually cut their lives short. What kind of lifestyle do they have?

Most diseases occur when there is a deficiency in minerals or vitamins in the body. Couple this with a lack of exercise and sleep, this deficiency starts to weakens parts of the body that eventually becomes diseased.

Acid reflux is one of the diseases that prevents certain minerals and vitamins from being absorbed into your body and, especially if you start taking drugstore or medical heartburn relievers that reduce the acid in your stomach.

Acid reflux doesn't happen when you eat a healthy diet. And, with a healthy diet, it doesn't mean a diet where you need to deprive yourself of the foods you like.

Most of us developed our eating habits from our parents. As we grew, we watched how they ate, when they ate, and what they ate. And, we did the same thing.

Stomach Acid

Acid reflux is not a problem of excess stomach acid or of stomach acid being too strong. Yet, all antacids and drugs are designed to decrease the strength of your stomach acid. When this is done, it is not a cure for your reflux, but just a temporary fix for your poor diet, eating habits, or lack of exercise.

What reflux drugs do is decrease the strength of your stomach acid, so when this acid goes up your esophagus, it will not affect your esophagus lining. The result is you will not feel heart burn or pain.

Acid Chamber

Your stomach was made to be an acid chamber. This means that your stomach acid needs to be around 1.0 to 3.0 pH, so that it can perform all the functions that it needs to.

When your stomach's pH moves above 3.0, your stomach automatically produces more acid to bring the pH down below 3.0.

When you take a drug to reduce your stomach acid and this acid pH moves above 3.0 pH, the digestion of your food will be compromised. There are many over the counter drugs that you can take without a doctor's prescription, but taking them can lead to dependence. Drugs can be used for immediate relief, but not for long term use. Long term use amplifies their side effects and leads to malnutrition.

As your stomach pH is maintain, around 3.0 or higher, your stomach acid is becoming more alkaline. Under these conditions your stomach acid pH will not burn your sensitive esophageal tissue. The result is you will not feel the burning sensation in chest area. This leads you to believe that you are cured, even though you may still have acid reflux. If you stop using the drug, the burning sensation may return and force you to continue using the reflux medication.

A Happy Stomach a Happy Person

Your stomach is happy and working like it should when its pH is 3.0 or less. Here are some of functions of your stomach:

1. break protein into its individual amino acids

2. prepare vitamins and minerals to be absorbed in the intestines

3. destroy incoming bacteria and pathogens

4. reduce chances of coming down with stomach cancer

5. keep stomach content acidic, so when it goes into the duodenum, it triggers pancreas digestive juices

6. reduce the chances of having allergies, skin disease, asthma, depression, lupus, grave's disease, osteoporosis, accelerated aging, and other conditions

In this book, you will find a new way of eating. Most of the problems that occur with eating are eating an acidic diet and overeating. Most people eat more than their body needs to keep them healthy and active.

The Acid Reflux Condition

Acid reflux occurs when stomach contents, which is acidic, flows into the esophagus and starts to burn the sensitive tissue there. This acid consists of Hydrochloric acid and pepsin, which is a digestive enzyme that digests protein and damages the esophageal tissue.

The acid burning is felt below the collar bone. Sometimes this burning or pain can be mistaken for heart pain. If this burning feeling only occurs occasionally, like once a month, then this is not a serious matter, which is easily corrected with information in this book.

Repeated acid reflux leads to damage to the esophagus lining. As this lining deteriorates, holes are created that form ulcers. These form the bases of Barrett's esophagus disease. Barrett's is the precursor to esophageal cancer. So, frequently bouts with acid reflux are not a condition to ignore.

Koufman Reflux Index

Below is a chart called the Koufman Reflux Symptom Index. You can take this quiz to determine if you have acid reflux. It's a chart that is useful to point out if you have Silent Reflux.

Many people are not even aware that they have issues with acid reflux. When you have silent acid reflux, you may never experience the typical heartburn symptom of full blow acid reflux. The big problem with silent reflux is it can damage your lungs, sinuses and throat, whereas your esophagus may not incur any damage.

Here's how to use Koufman's Reflux Index. Look at each question and determine the level, from 0 to 5, whether the symptom pertains to you.

A score of 15 or more indicates you might have a 90% chance of having acid reflux. Check the search engine, if you want a downloadable print of this chart.

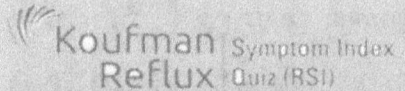

Koufman Symptom Index
Reflux Quiz (RSI)

Within the last MONTH, how did the following problems affect you?	0 = No Problem 5 = Severe Problem					
Hoarseness or a problem with your voice	0	1	2	3	4	5
Clearing your throat	0	1	2	3	4	5
Excess throat mucous or postnasal drip	0	1	2	3	4	5
Difficulty swallowing food, liquids, or pills	0	1	2	3	4	5
Coughing after you ate or after lying down	0	1	2	3	4	5
Breathing difficulties or choking episodes	0	1	2	3	4	5
Troublesome or annoying cough	0	1	2	3	4	5
Sensations of something sticking in your throat or a lump in your throat	0	1	2	3	4	5
Heartburn, chest pain, indigestion, or stomach acid coming up	0	1	2	3	4	5

Your RSI is

2: Lower Esophagus Sphincter, LES

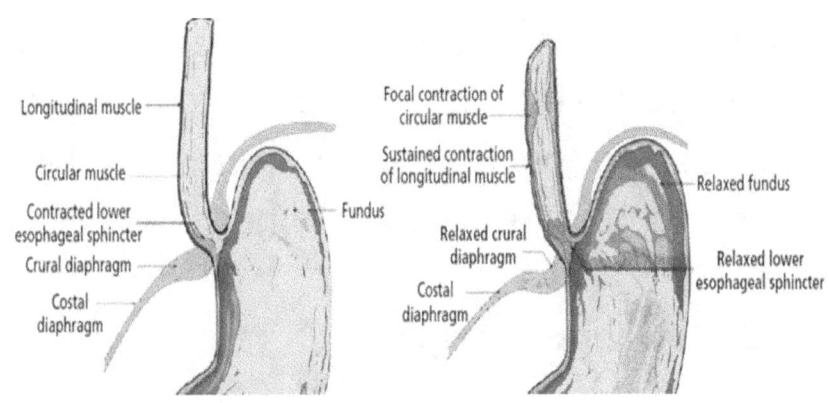

Two Esophagus Sphincters

The esophagus maintains movement of food by two sphincters. It has an upper sphincter, close to your throat, that opens in responds to your swallowing food. Then, it passes food down your esophagus toward the lower esophagus sphincter. It takes 4 to 8 seconds for food to move from your throat to your stomach. It takes even less when you drink something.

The movement of food along the esophagus is so strong that even when you are upside down, food will still reach your stomach.

The lower esophagus sphincter is a gate way into your stomach. It opens to let food in and closes to prevent food from re-entering your esophagus from your stomach.

The Crural Diaphragm

The lower sphincter is a muscle, which closes and opens with the help of the crural diaphragm. The crural diaphragm is a tissue that separates the abdomen from your chest area. The lower sphincter passes through the diaphragm, which puts external pressure on the sphincter to close or open when necessary.

Stomach Gas Pressure

When you have a weak LES, the gas

pressure from your stomach will easily open your LES, allowing food to flow back into your esophagus. This gas can become excessive when you eat a poor combination of food, eat too much food, drink too much liquid during your meal, or eat fruit or a sugary desert after your meal.

But, a low tone LES is not always the reason that you might have acid reflux, because there are many other factors that contributes to acid reflux.

However, research has shown that you can have acid reflux even when you have a normal LES strength. But, studies are ongoing to try to find drugs that will strengthen the LES in people with acid reflux.

3: Medication You Can
for Acid Reflux

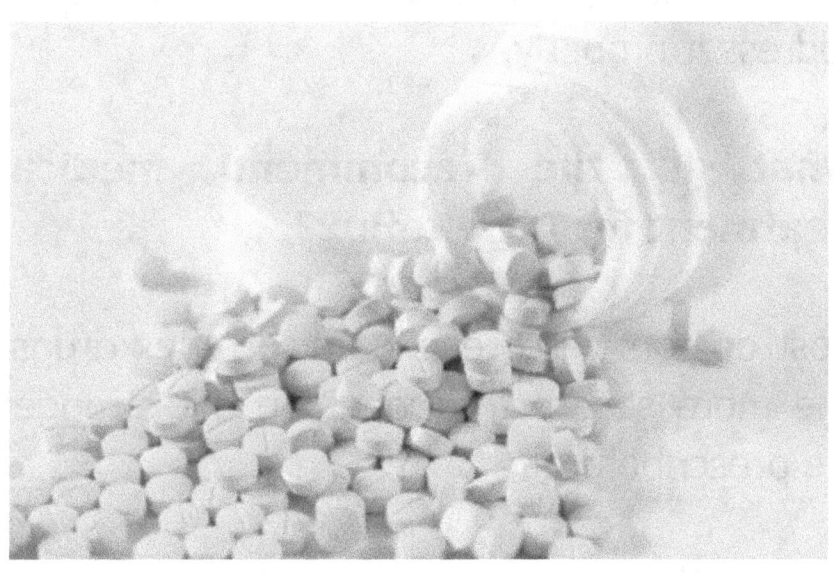

There are many over the counter drugs for acid reflux that you can buy. There are also many drugs that are only available through your doctor's prescription. What you do to handle your acid reflux or GERD will be your decision. This decision will determine the future of your health.

In this chapter, you will find information that will help you decide if you want to use drugs or not. It is recommended that if you have a severe case of acid reflux, GERD, that you see your doctor. Continual acid reflux has some serious consequents, if you do not address it properly.

What is the recommend medical treatment for Acid Reflux?

Most doctors will prescribe acid reflux drugs. The more severe the condition the stronger the prescribe drug.

Acid Reflux Drugs

- antacids
- H2 blockers
- proton-pump inhibitors (PPIs)
- histamine-2 blockers
- Alginate
- LES inhibitors

Antacids

Antacids are available at your corner drugstore, OTC. However, many people might use baking soda and water as a quick fix for their reflux, before they head to a drug store. But, it is not a good idea to frequently use this home remedy, when you have acid reflux.

These antacids or OTC's are designed to neutralize or block the formation of stomach acid, causing its pH to go above 3.0. As the acid pH moves up to 4 and higher, it is becoming more alkaline. Under these conditions it will not burn your sensitive esophageal tissue and you will not feel the burning sensation. This leads you to believe that you are cured, but you may have to continue using the drug to feel cured.

These OTC's come in tablet and liquid form. Since there are many brands that target the reduction of stomach acid, you may be confused as to which one to buy.

These Antacids can provide quick short term relief and should not be used for over a week. One of the draw backs of using these antacids for long term is they interfere with your nutrient creation and absorption and can lead to nutrient deficiencies.

You will find that these OTC's contain,

- calcium cargonate
- aluminum hydroxide
- sodium bicarbonate
- magnesium hydroxide

H2 Blockers

Some of the H2 blockers are,

Pepcid AC

Tagamet and Zantac 75 (ranitidine)

Cimetidine

Famotidine

These H-2-receptor block the stomach cells production of stomach acid for up to 12 hours. They are available over the counter or in prescription.

Proton-pump inhibitors (PPIs)

Proton-pump inhibitors, PPIs, are stronger than H-2-receptor blockers. They reduce acid production by your stomach walls and do this longer than the H2 blockers. This gives your esophageal tissue relief and time to heal.

They also are available over the counter or by prescription.

The PP's include:

Omeprazole

Rabeprazole

Nexium (esomeprazole)

Preyacid

Prilosec

AcipHex

Protonix

At times a doctor may prescribe a drug called prokinetic agents to be taken with PPI's. These drugs activate the stomach to release its contents into the duodenum quicker than normal.

Histamine-2 blockers

Histamine-2 blockers also block HCL acid secretions from your stomach lining.

Alginate drugs

Alginate drugs are a different composition than other antacids. These drugs do contain an antacid, but have a different action in the stomach than a typical antacid.

Alginate comes from a water-soluble seaweed fiber.

Alginate drugs work through the action of their ingredient alginic acid. This acid works by forming a mechanical barrier against your stomach acid near the top of your stomach and LES. This prevents stomach acid from moving into your esophagus and causing damage. And, at the same time, it has no effect on the pH of your stomach acid.

Gaviscon is one of most frequently used alginate drug for acid reflux or heartburn. It coats the esophagus lining and the upper stomach, which prevents reflux.

The active ingredient in alginate drugs, alginic acid, is found in brown algae.

LES inhibitors

LES inhibitors prevent the lower esophageal valve from relaxing. In some cases of reflux, the LES tends to relax after eating. When this happens, acid reflux is more likely to occur.

Other Acid Reflux Options

Here is a list of other reflux options that might be taken by your doctor.

- Sucralfate acid suppressants
- Transient lower esophageal sphincter relaxation (TLESR) reducers
- GABA(B) receptor agents
- mGluR5 antagonist
- Prokinetic agents
- Pain modulators
- Tricyclic antidepressants
- Selective <u>serotonin</u> reuptake inhibitors (SSRIs)
- Antihistamines
- Sedatives
- Painkillers
- antidepressants

Side effects of Acid Reflux Drugs

Research done in various clinical studies show that most acid reflux drug, when used frequently or for a long time, have side effects such as:

- Kidney damage
- Increased bone fractures
- Contributor to dementia
- Increased risk for heart arrhythmias, osteoporosis, and bacterial pneumonia
- Increased risk for nutritional deficiencies and intestinal infections

In a serious study done at Washington University School of Medicine, St. Louis, it was found the proton pump inhibitors increased your risk of premature death.

Effects of Acid Reflux Drugs

Doctors will always recommend PPI's or H2

blockers, if you have acid reflux or GERD. Since, these drugs reduce stomach acid; they are effective in protecting your esophagus. Because of their side effects, it is important to use these medications for a limited time.

Using acid reflux drugs becomes necessary, at times, to prevent tissue damage in your esophagus and the resulting heartburn. Frequent bouts with reflux can lead to complication such as Barrett's esophagus and esophageal cancer.

Some doctors recommend using reflux drugs for up to 8 weeks. In this ebook, you will find many natural remedies that will help you fix your acid reflux. That way you don't become dependent on drugs to keep you free of heartburn and stomach discomfort.

Use of antacids and acid reflux and OTC medication when used for a long time, one year or longer, were found to lead to heart attacks, dementia, liver failure, other diseases and premature death.

Not Responding to Drugs

Some people with reflux or GERD may not respond to the use of drugs. Some of these cases may involve people, who are obese, have anemia, liver issues, problems swallowing, or other physical ailments.

In these cases, it is best to work with your doctor so various tests can be performed to determine the severity of your reflux condition.

4: Discover Details about Heartburn, Acid Reflux, GERD?

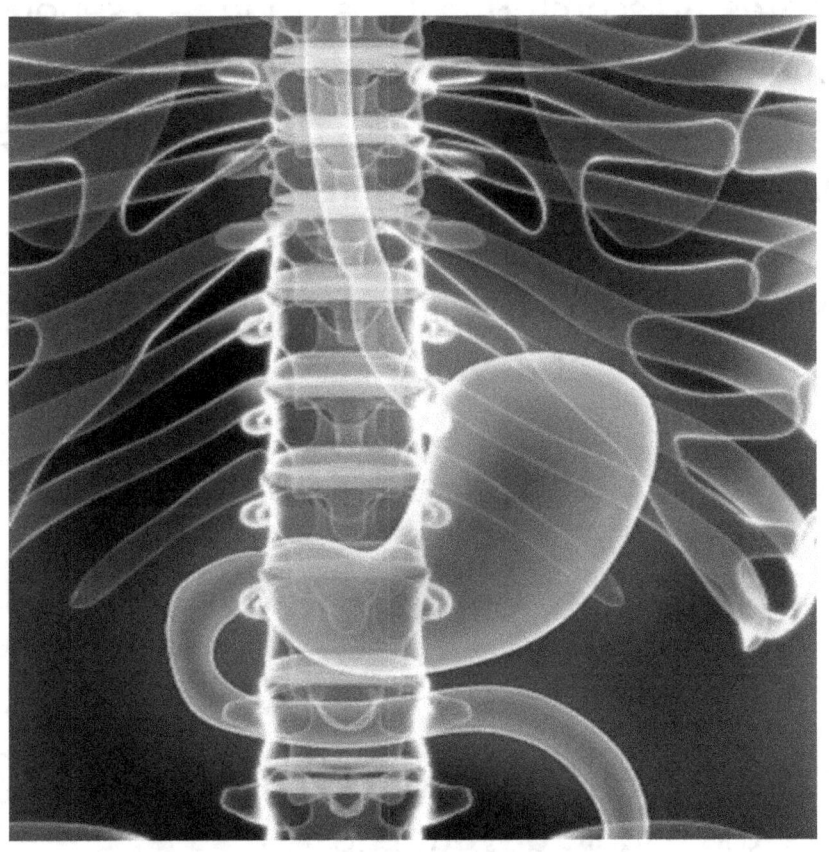

Acid reflux is the condition where stomach acid has pushed through your LES and into your esophagus.   Heartburn is a symptom created by acid reflux where you feel a burning sensation in the lower chest. The burning is a result of acid attacking the lining your esophagus.

Although heartburn can be painful and creates discomfort, it is not a serious condition provided it does not occur too frequently.   This type of condition can be managed by using natural remedies.

Acid reflux is not limited to specific ages, but can occur at any age.

Typical Heartburn Symptoms

- Bad, sour, or bitter taste or in your mouth
- Burning feeling from the below throat to the middle of your chest
- Burping
- Difficulty swallowing or pain when

swallowing

- A feeling of fullness
- Pain develops 30-60 minutes after eating and last for hour
- Dental erosion
- Sore or hoarse throat
- Vomiting
- Wheezing
- Persistent cough
- Abdominal pain or cramps

What Causes Acid Reflux, Silent Acid Reflux, GERD, or Heartburn?

Acid reflux or GERD and the symptom heartburn occur when the esophagus valve opens and allows acid to "reflux" or move up into your esophagus, where it burns your sensitive tissue.

Acid reflux is not caused by excess

stomach acid, as is promoted by the medical community. The major cause is poor eating habits or a weak or faulty lower esophageal sphincter, LES, which allows stomach acid back into an area where it does not belong.

Acid reflux is also caused by eating too much food or eating a combination of foods that does not mix well. When this happen, your food will not digest properly, causing gas to build up in your stomach and forcing your LES valve to open. With your LES valve open, your stomach gas forces some of the acidic content to move back into your esophagus.

Now the question arises, if you use drugstore acid reducers will you get relief from acid reflux or heartburn. Yes you will, by reducing your stomach acid strength, you will not burn your esophagus tissue as much, but it is not a cure for your acid reflux or GERD. And, the continual use of these products will cause you some serious health issue.

Cause of Acid Reflux and GERD

GERD is a serious case of acid reflux. Its causes are the same acid reflux. Here are lists of foods that may give rise to your acid reflux. Not everyone is affected by these foods, since each one is a different person and has a different lifestyle history.

One of the main causes of reflux is overeating. Other causes that make you prone to reflux are:

- Hiatus hernia
- Poor diet, low fiber, fatty food
- Obesity
- Alcohol
- Coffee or caffeinated drinks
- Smoking
- Chocolate,

- Sodas
- Fried, citrus, spicy foods
- Tomatoes and their sauces
- Garlic, onions
- Mint
- Lack of exercise
- Use of prescribed drugs, antidepressants, progesterone
- Posture
- Pregnancy

Silent Acid Reflux

Silent acid reflux, also known as **laryngeal pharyngeal reflux,** is a condition where you can have acid reflux and don't know it. The symptoms that you may experience are more subtle than full blown acid reflux. The result is these subtle symptoms may appear to belong to some other condition.

Because stomach content that moves into your esophagus can push into your throat, it can also get into your ears, nose, sinuses, lungs, mouth, vocal cords, and ears. When this happens, you can get symptoms that appear not related to acid reflux.

The most common symptoms of silent reflux are:

- Difficulty swallowing
- Snoring
- Bad breath
- Chronic cough
- Sinusitis
- Post-nasal drip
- Hoarseness
- Asthma
- Tooth decay
- Sleep apnea
- Sore throat

Coughing can be associated with silent acid reflux. If stomach content moves into your throat, it can cause tiny droplets of stomach acid to drop onto your throat. This can cause hoarseness, coughing, throat irritation, and throat clearing.

Making Heartburn Worse

The following activities can make your heartburn worst, but are not the cause of it.

Lying down flat causes your stomach to press down on your LES. If your LES is weak, acid will flow back up into your esophagus. By raising your head, when you lie down, you can move your esophagus higher than your stomach. This makes it more difficult for acid to flow into your esophagus. Wait at least 2 hours before lying down, after a meal.

After eating, tight clothes, belts, stooping, and bending can squeeze your stomach, pushing up acid food into your esophagus. .

OTC Remedies

Simple remedies to use for quick reflux relief consist of using **OTC acid blockers**. These blockers my contain calcium or magnesium. As with any acid blockers, their use should not exceed one to two weeks.

Alginate, when used in an antacid, has shown to be more effective than just using OTC antacids.   Look for an alginate OTC when dealing with an infrequent reflux problem. **Gaviscon** is one of most frequently used alginate drug for acid reflux or heartburn.

Asthma

Acid reflux can be misdiagnosed as asthma. When you have acid reflux, you may have trouble breathing.   When you have asthma, you have trouble getting air from your lungs.

But with acid reflux you can have trouble getting air into your body.

5: Dealing with Acid Reflux During Pregnancy

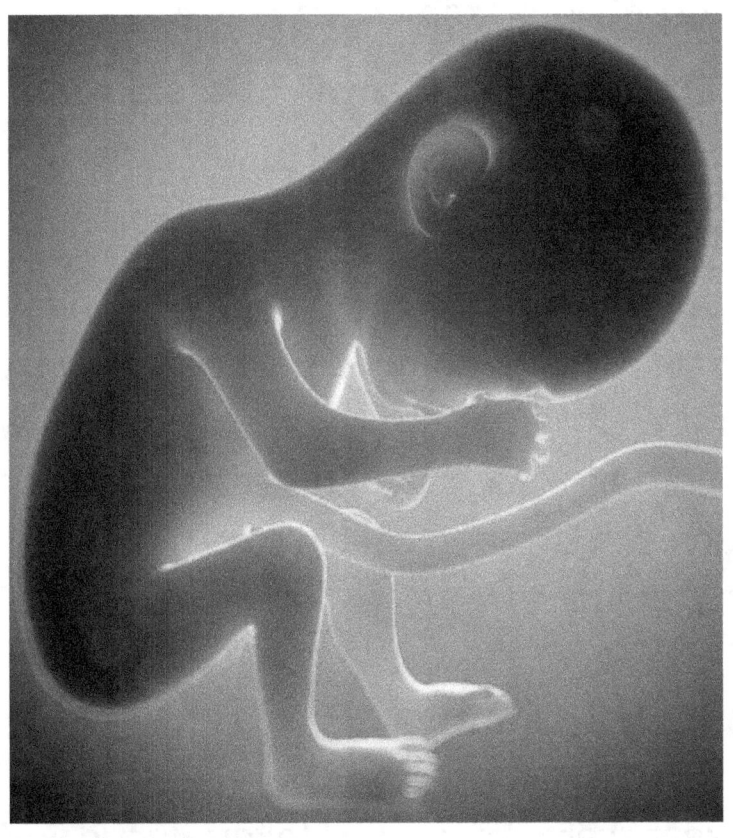

Most women experience acid reflux during pregnancy and suffer from heartburn and indigestion. This is due to the baby pushing against the stomach and LES. However, there are many other conditions and lifestyle choices that result in acid reflux in pregnancy, such as:

- Increase estrogen and progesterone which can lead to relaxation of the lower esophageal sphincter

- Increase pressure on the stomach with growing uterus

As outline in other chapters, following many of the recommendations can help you minimize or eliminate your experience with acid reflux. By experimenting with the various diet and remedies listed, you can find which one gives you the best relief.

Using Medication

Great care must be taken when using antacids or medication to deal with acid reflux. These mediations decrease the strength of your stomach acid and interfere with the creation and absorption of vitamins and minerals.

Here is recap of some of the ideas to avoid acid reflux:

- Eat small meals throughout the day.
- Do not lie down until one hour or more after eating
- Avoid eating those foods that you find give you acid reflux
- Before eating, eat a small amount of yogurt or milk with honey
- Do regular gentle exercise
- Improve diet
- Avoid eating late at night. Try eating last meal 3 hours before bed time.

Antacids

It is best to always talk to your doctor before using any medication, including antacids. If you take iron supplements, antacids will interfere with their absorption.

Antacids are considered safe for most people, but it is best **not to use them during your pregnancy**. Antacids give quick relief for heartburn, but it is better to get to the cause of heartburn and reduce it.

Sodium Bicarbonate

Sodium bicarbonate should not be used at any time during your pregnancy because of side effects for you and your baby.

Histamine2-receptor antagonists

This drug has been used by many pregnant women and has not shown any damage or harm to a fetus. Histamine2 drugs are cimetidine, ranitidine, famotidine. The drug **nizatidine** has shown frequent fetal damage in animals. Always, talk to your doctor before taking acid reflux OTC drugs.

It is always best to avoid OTC drugs, because, side effects are not always know in the long term. It's better to use food as a way to decrease or eliminate acid reflux.

Proton pump inhibitors (PPIs)

These inhibitors have limited safety information for pregnant women. The drug **omeprazole** should not be used since it may cause harmful effects on your fetus.

Some doctors might prescribe PPIs in severe cases of acid reflux, as a last resort.

6: Natural Lifestyle and Acid Reflux Diet

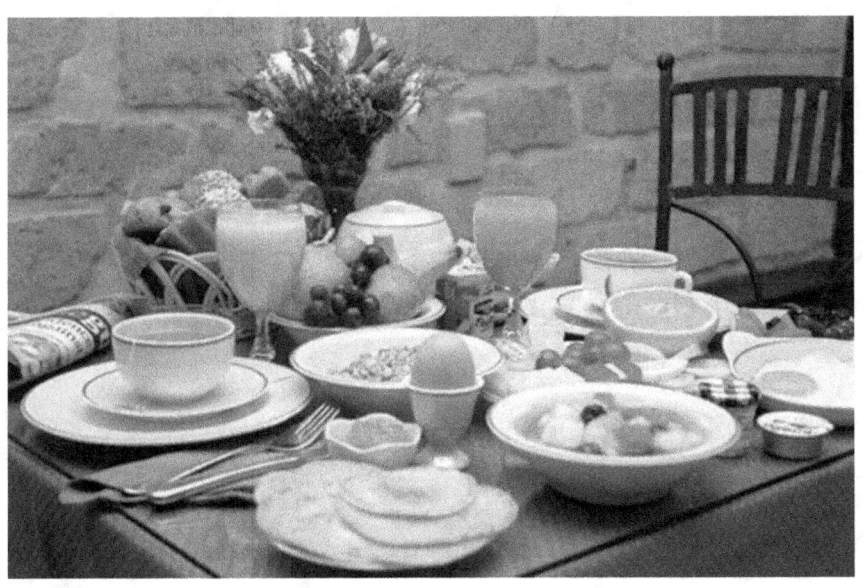

The natural lifestyle and diet for eliminating heartburn or acid reflux is to:

1. stop doing and eating the things that promote acid reflux

2. start doing the things that help eliminate acid reflux

3. Start using natural remedies that will help to strengthen or normalize your stomach and lower esophageal sphincter, LES.
4. Start using supplements that strengthen all the tissues in your body.

Studies have shown that eating a good diet and combining food properly can replace the use of drugs for reflux.

Here is a list of what you can do to live a healthier lifestyle to make sure acid reflux does not turn into a damaging disease. The list below can be done little by little. The most important first steps will be pointed out.

- Follow a healthy diet
- If overweight, lose some overweight
- Decrease exposure to toxins
- Detox your body daily
- Maintain some daily exercise

- Maintain 8 to 9 hours of sleep
- Have Daily activities
- Reduce stress
- Choose natural acid reflux remedies
- Keep a schedule of taking supplements
- Develop good gut health

HCL Pills

One of the secrets in controlling and eliminating heartburn and acid reflux is to take HCl acid pills. Heartburn often occurs not because of excess acid in the stomach, but because of not enough acid. But, taking HCl pills should be done under the direction of your doctor. If you want to add HCL to your supplements, get the digestive enzyme supplements that contain HCL.

Your stomach is your first line of good health. Keeping your stomach working right will insure that you will get the right nutrition into your blood.

Keeping a Happy Stomach

Here is a list of eating rules that you need to follow to be heartburn free or if you just want to be free of having digestive problems.

Digestive Enzymes

Just before you eat, take 2 digestive enzymes to help you digest your food. You don't want undigested food to go into your colon, especially meat. Undigested meat is one of the causes of colon cancer, constipation, diverticulitis, and other colon issues.

Eating slowly allows your stomach to digest your food better and quicker. Food digestion starts in your mouth and the more you chew your food the more it prepares it for your stomach to complete the job.

Over eating can cause acid reflux. When you over eat, the LES may not close properly or may open easily to let acid back into your esophagus.

Drinking Liquids

Limit the amount of liquid you drink when you eat. This dilutes the acid in your stomach that you need to digest your food. If you do drink liquid, use room temperature water, since cold water slows down your digestive process. But, drink water only to clear your throat.

Eating Sugar

Limit your consumption of sugar when you eat. Sugar has no nutritional value and causes calcium to get expelled in your urine. In addition, other minerals are used up during its digestion. For sure don't drink soda or other sweet drinks during your meals.

After you eat, don't eat any fruit. Your stomach is busy digesting the food you just ate. Eating fruit will cause the fruit to remain in your stomach waiting to be digested and will start fermenting and decaying causing gas and pain.

Salt

Limit your use of salt during meals since it also affects your calcium absorption. You can eat salty treats between meals.

Food Digestion

Limit the food that you eat. When you eat excess food where you combine meat, carbohydrates, sugar, sodas, fats, and processed foods, your stomach cannot properly digest them and turns them into toxic acids. This acid creates gas and can put pressure on a weak LES, causing it to open.

Eating mostly acid food usually causes a weak LES, which can open during your digestion process. A balanced diet, which contains both acid and alkaline foods, keeps your LES strong and will not open, when you occasionally eat more food than you should.

There are certain foods that cause more stomach problems than others. For this reason, you should minimize eating these foods.

Protein

Protein and bread are considered an acid food. Start Eating less protein and bread. Protein stays in your stomach up to 4 hours, since it takes a long time to digest. If you don't have enough stomach acid, some of the protein you eat will not get digested. To maintain a healthy stomach function all of your food in your stomach must be digested properly.

Guess who likes it when you don't digest your protein very good, the bad bacteria in your colon. They thrive on undigested protein. When your bad bacteria thrive in your colon, your colon doesn't work right.

How to Eat Protein

If you don't eat vegetables with your protein, this is a big problem. Your protein is going to take a long time going through your colon, or in other words, you will be constipation. When you are constipated and you eat your next meal, there will be pressure on your stomach from your colon and your stomach digestion will be delayed.

So, eat smaller protein portions and always eat them with raw or slightly cooked vegetables. Vegetables provide fiber, which mixes with the digested protein providing quicker digestion of protein. Don't eat fruit with your meals or as desert. This slows down the digestion of your protein. Wait about 1 1/2 after your meal, before you eat desert.

If you cook your vegetables, some of the fiber is neutralized and you don't get the full benefit of raw fiber in your colon.

How to Eat Bread

Now, the same is true about bread or other flour products. They digest quicker than protein in the stomach, but in the colon they move very slowly. In your colon flour products are like dough and this makes it hard to move them with peristaltic movements. Again, eat them with vegetables unless you want to be constipated.

When's the Best Time to Eat Protein and Carbohydrates

Now, here is the best time and way to eat protein and carbohydrates. At lunch or dinner only eat one or the other with raw vegetables. If you can, eat protein and vegetables and no carbohydrates. Or, eat carbohydrates and vegetables and no protein.

Eating in this way is based on your body cycles. In the next chapter, you will be introduced to eating with your body cycles. This is the best way to eliminate acid reflux. It is also the best way to eat, which will result in you having good stomach function.

7: Fiber for Your Acid Reflux

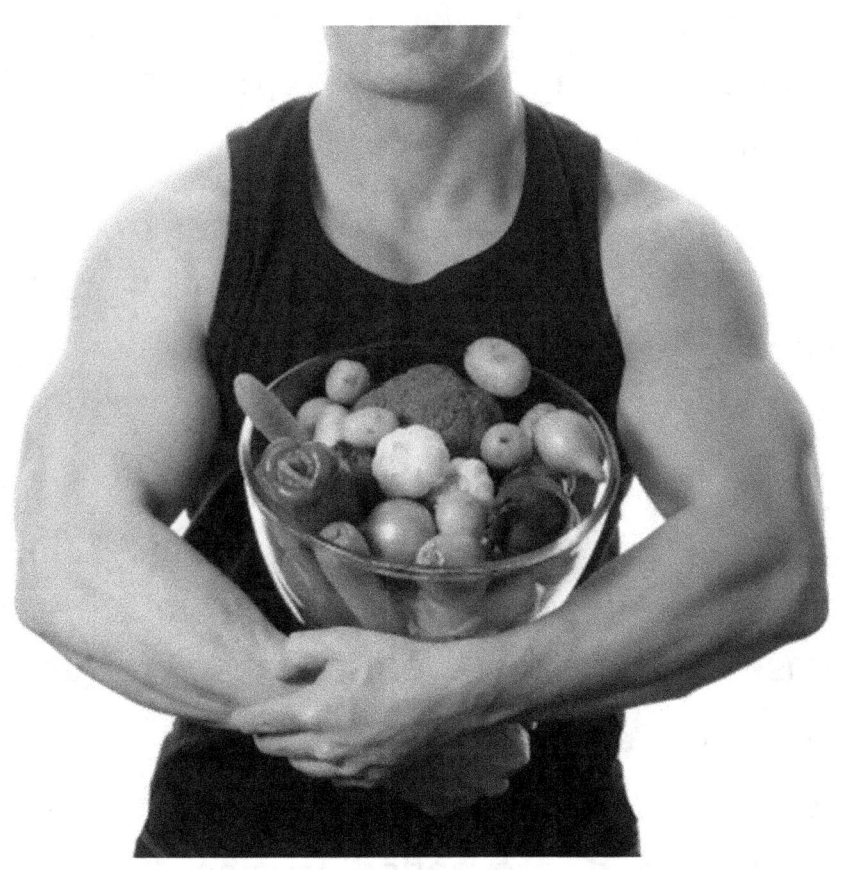

What is Fiber?

One of the main reasons you might have acid reflux is that you don't have enough fiber in your diet. Fiber is a necessary substance that prevents you from having constipation. When you have frequent constipation and you strain to have a bowel movement, you put pressure on the top of your stomach and LES. This can force your LES to open.

Fiber is a carbohydrate that comes from the cell's walls and structure of plants, grains, legumes, fruits, and vegetables. Most processed or junk food has little or no fiber, since it was removed during processing.

Most people eat around 7-12 grams of fiber each day. You should be eating from 25 – 40 grams each day to prevent serious illnesses in your body.

A diet with 40 grams of fiber provides protection and prevention against diseases such as acid reflux, kidney stones, varicose veins, obesity, heart disease, appendicitis, colon disease, diabetes, appendicitis, diverticulosis, and hiatus hernia.

It will be difficult for you to reach 40 grams of fiber a day, if you are not eating very many fruits and vegetables. You have to start adding produce to your diet slowly, so that you will not experience excessive fiber side effects.

When you eat fiber, it passes into your colon without getting digested in the small intestine. The good bacteria will use some of it as food, which makes them stronger and able to multiply.

Eating fiber reduces your fecal matter transit time from three days to 1 1/ 2 - 2days.

All processed foods, such as white flour products, have little or no fiber. Fiber is removed when various natural flours or grains are processed to make junk food. During this processing, nutrients, vitamins, and minerals are also removed. Only plant foods and lightly processed grains have fiber of varying amounts.

Soluble Fiber

Soluble Fiber becomes gummy and viscous, after it dissolves in water. Soluble fiber can slow down digestion in the small intestine and prevent simple sugars from entering the bloodstream right away. Because it absorbs water, soluble fiber softens and gives weight to fecal matter, and this makes fecal matter easier to pass through your colon.

Soluble fiber consists of pectin, gum, and mucilage. Pectin is found in carrots, apples, beets, cabbage, citrus fruits, and bananas. Gums and mucilage are found in oat bran, sesame seeds, oats, oatmeal, legumes, guar gum, and gum Arabic

Insoluble Fiber

Insoluble fiber does not dissolve in water and consists of cellulose, hemi cellulose, and lignin. This type of fiber is extremely beneficial to your health. Because your body's enzymes cannot break down, this fiber remains in tack as it travels through your intestines and colon.

Insoluble fiber helps fecal matter travel faster through the small intestine and your colon. It provides bulk to your fecal matter. It makes your stools larger, softer, and stimulates peristaltic movement, as it touches your colon walls.

Insoluble fibers are found in vegetables, wheat, and wheat bran. This type of fiber is considered an anti-carcinogen and a digestive aid. It is credited with preventing colon cancer and many other colon diseases.

Eating Fiber

As you can see, fiber is a critical nutrient for your overall health. You need to eat equal amounts of insoluble and soluble fiber. Most people only eat around 10 grams or less of fiber each day. The amount you need to eat is around 25 – 40 grams. This is a lot of fiber, and you will need to introduce it slowly into your diet. You may experience gas when you eat more fiber than you normally do.

Health Alert: If you have any serious gastrointestinal illnesses, check with your doctor before adding more fiber to your diet.

If you have not been eating a lot of fiber in the form of vegetable, fruits, and grains, you need to add these foods to your eating habits little by little, so your body gets use to more fiber.

Health Tip: Provide yourself with natural forms of fiber, such as vegetables, fruits, and legumes. Stay away from the supplemental forms of fiber such as, powders or pills that may help in relieving constipation, but do little to provide you with other nutrients those natural forms of fiber provide.

Eating Bran

Eating bran is one of the quickest and best ways to increase your fiber. It will increase the weight and size of your stools more than the fiber contained in fruits or vegetables.

Bran is the outer husk of the grain – wheat, corn, rice, and oat – which is indigestible.

Use one or two heaping tablespoon of bran in your morning cereal, in your baking, and in your smoothies.

Health Alert: When using bran, make sure you drink plenty of water during the day to keep your stools soft.

There are four basic bran products – wheat, corn, oat, and rice. They all provide a solid source of fiber in varying amounts. Make sure the bran you use is 100% unprocessed bran. Here are the two recommended bran products.

Oat Bran

Oat bran has both soluble and insoluble fiber, which make its better to use than wheat bran. However, it does have less insoluble fiber than wheat and rice bran. It can be found with relatively little processing, which helps to maintain its high quality of protein, carbohydrates and vitamins.

Rice Bran

For preventing constipation, rice bran is better than wheat bran. Do not take your calcium supplement with bran cereals, since fiber can interfere with calcium absorption.

Do not use cereal with bran in it. This bran has been processed and has lost some of its fiber content. Use the bran sold as coarse granules. Add it to your morning cereals, smoothies, shakes, cottage cheese, yogurt, or other dishes.

Sources of Insoluble Fiber

- Bananas
- Broccoli
- Brown rice
- Brussels sprouts
- Cauliflower
- Cabbage
- Corn
- Lentils

- Potatoes

- Spinach wheat germ

- Whole wheat bread

- Whole wheat crackers

Sources of Soluble Fiber

- Oranges, grapefruit, nectarines, peaches, tangerines, apples, berries, apricots, bananas, figs, prunes

- Zucchini, turnips, okra, cabbage, peas, sweet potatoes

- Carrots, celery, broccoli, cauliflower, corn, eggplant, okra, Zucchini, greens

- Barley, chickpeas, split peas, pinto beans, kidney beans, navy beans, potatoes

8: Eating Body Cycles That Eliminate Acid Reflux

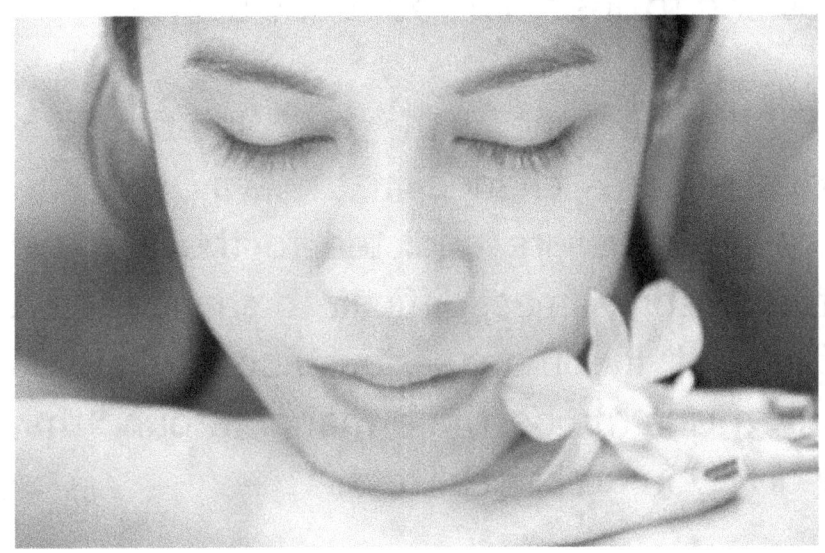

Natural Body Cycles

Most of you are looking for ways to get rid constipation, improve your health, or lose weight and of course acid reflux. Here's some information that will help you achieve these results. It's called "Using the Natural Body Cycles" for achieving maximum health.

By learning how to assist your "Natural Body Cycles", you will be in tune with what your body is doing to properly digest your food. You will be in tune on how to eliminate acids and toxins from your body daily.

Getting in tune with your Natural Body Cycles requires change in the way you eat. Since all of us are addicted to the way we eat, it is, sometimes, difficult to change these habits. But, if you are serious about what you want, this is the best information around that will give you great health.

By using this method to gain better body health, you may experience some side effects because you will be eliminating more body toxins and body wastes. The side effects maybe headaches, stomach upsets or body pain. These conditions will not last and will disappear as you get rid of more and more toxins. So if you experience these side effects, don't let them stop you from moving forward in this eating pattern.

Here are the 3 natural body cycles:

Cycle 1 time period: 4 a.m. to 12 noon

This cycle is the time where your body is eliminating toxins, acids, wastes, and derby by urine, bowel movements, and other secretions. Most people interfere with this cycle, since they are unaware of it, causing constipation and various detrimental illnesses.

Cycle 2 time period: 12 noon to 8 p.m.

This is the time when your body should be taking in food and digesting it. By eating the right kind of food at the right time, you help your digestive process in your stomach and small intestine.

Cycle 3 time period: 8 p.m. to 4 a.m.

This is the time your body is absorbing

and using the food you have eaten from 12 noon to 8 p.m.

The First Body Cycle

During the elimination cycle, 4 a.m. to 12 noon, eat only fruits and vegetables and their juices. For breakfast, eat a bowl of fruit or have a fruit smoothie made with apple juice, banana, and fruits in season.

Before noontime eat fruits as a snack.

Forty-five minutes before noon eat your last fruit. You can eat and drink all the fruits and juices you want up to noontime.

If you like oats eat them, but only unprocessed oats. Vary the days that you eat them. You can add the fruits that you like to them.

Fruits are made by nature and are the perfect food. They contain the right balance of nutrients with about 70% distilled water. You gain enormous benefits from eating fruits, especially if you eat the outer skin. Eat them without cooking them. They are easy to digest and absorb and do not stress your stomach, small intestine, or colon. They activate peristaltic action in your colon and help you have a bowel movement to excrete toxins.

Here are some of the fruits to eat:

Watermelons

Apples

Apricots

Avocados

Bananas

Blueberries

Boysenberries

Cantaloupes

Cherries

Figs and dates

Grapes

Grapes

Lemons

Nectarines

Oranges

Papayas

Peaches

Pears

Persimmons

Plums

Prunes

Raspberries

Strawberries

Eat all melons together and not with other fruit. Wait 1/2 hour before eating other fruits. Melons require specific enzymes to be digested in the stomach, so other fruit eaten with melons will just sit in your stomach, waiting to be digested and can cause gas and belching.

By eating fruits during body cycle 1, you are assisting your body's elimination cycle. This helps your body to have bowel movements and urinate. This also helps you eliminate toxins and acids from your body and blood. It is these toxins and acids that make you sick, overweight, constipated. They weaken your LES and can lead to acid reflux.

Eating solid food for breakfast – eggs potatoes, rice, meat, box cereal, milk, and so on, the typical breakfast, interferes with your body's elimination cycle and eventually leads to sickness and excess weight.

It takes over 3 hours to digest heavy and solid food. The food you should be eating in the morning should digest quickly to help activate peristaltic colon action to help you have a bowel movement and to continue your body's nightly detoxification process.

A morning heavy breakfast slows down your elimination of toxins from your body. This causes fecal matter to remain in your colon longer than it should. Toxins in the fecal matter can be reabsorbed into your body. These toxins then get stored in your body as fat and acids. An acid body is one of the main causes of most illnesses.

You need an alkaline body to have the best health possible. Fruits and vegetables neutralize acids and give you an alkaline body. An alkaline body is the healthiest body condition you can have.

It takes ½ to 1 hour or so to digest fruits and fruit and vegetable juices. Because of this, they help to cleanse your body of waste during the time from 4am to noontime. Fruits are 70% water, just like your body, and this gives them the cleansing action they have and that your body needs.

So if you are not already having fruit and fruit and vegetables juices for breakfast and snacks, start slowing changing your habits, if you want to lose weight and feel better.

Now, one other thing, don't eat fruits and juices after your lunch or dinner. Wait at least 1 to 1 ½ hours after your meals before eating fruit snacks.

The Second Natural Body Cycle

Here is the second body cycle and it occurs from 12 noon to 8 p.m.

This is the time when your body should be taking in solid food and digesting it. What you eat has to be in alignment with what your stomach can do.

Here's how your stomach works. In

generally it can only digest one solid food at a time.

A solid food is one that does not contain 70% water, like fruits and vegetables do. It is a food that has been cooked, baked, or microwaved.

Your stomach can only work on one solid food at a time, so your lunch and dinner should only have one solid food. A lunch can consist of:

- chicken a green salad
- fish a green salad
- tuna and a green salad
- shrimp and a green salad
- beef and a green salad
- hard boiled eggs a salad
- beans and a salad

Eat in this fashion until your digestion starts to improve, and you start to get some relief from acid reflux.

Mixing a protein meal with carbohydrates is giving the stomach two solid foods at the same time. This causes the carbohydrate to sit in the stomach until the protein is digested. This will cause gas and increase stomach pressure, which can lead to reflux. If you want to eat a carbohydrate with meat don't eat as much of it as you normally do.

Giving the stomach more than it can handle interrupts the elimination cycle 1, and reduces the energy that you need for the elimination cycle, for the next day.

Any eating habit that disrupts cycle 2, the eating and digestion cycle, affects the other cycles. Here's how you can help your body's cycle 2 to be more effective. By doing these things, you can reduce that potential of acid reflux.

1. Eat only one solid food with vegetables during lunch or dinner. Lunch can be one meat or seafood with a fresh vegetable

salad.

2. Limit the amount of water you drink during meals. Drinking excess water will dilute your digestive acids and slow down the digestion of your food.

3. Avoid drinking sodas, tea or other drinks during your meals. If you need to clear your dry throat, use room temperature water. Cold liquids will slow down your digestive processes.

4. Eating meals with more than one solid food such as meat and potatoes, chicken and rice, fish and rice, chicken and noodles, eggs and toast, cheese and bread will diminish the energy you need during the elimination cycle. In addition, it will be more difficult to digest your food causing excess gas to be created.

5. It is permissible to eat beef and chicken at the same time but not chicken and eggs or

beef and nuts or chicken and beans. Eat the same type of protein at the same time, but do not mix different proteins.

6. It's ok to eat different types of carbohydrates at the same time, with a salad, but not with protein, since carbohydrates digest easier than protein.

Eating a protein and a carbohydrate at the same time sets the stage for severe illness later in life. A protein requires acid for digestion, and a carbohydrate requires alkaline juices for digestion. This combination produces acid juices and alkaline juices at the same time. This combination produces water, which creates digestive juices that cannot fully digest either type of food.

In this case, the body produces more acid and more alkaline juices, which again are neutralized. This cycle continues until the food in your stomach starts to putrefy and ferment causing gas and acids. The gas causes belching and the combination of gas and acids can lead to acid reflux.

As foods turns into acids because of putrefaction and the fermentation process, this acid food spoils all of the food in your stomach, causing undigested food to back flow into your esophagus and flow prematurely into your small intestine.

Food that is partially undigested becomes acidic, which affect the health of your colon and cause constipation. When these acids are absorbed into your body, they are converted into fat and stored as acid toxins your body.

In many cases, the fermentation of food results in the production of alcohol and is similar to a person who drinks alcohol. There have been cases where people have been arrested for drunk driving and have never drank in the life, and they wonder why they had a high blood alcohol level.

Eating the right combination of foods at meal time helps to preserve your energy for the elimination cycle. And, it prevents you from creating spoiled food in your stomach that is converted to acid waste. It is this acid waste that results in illness and fat. This is the reason most people, as they age, show various illnesses that have been developing over time. .

The Third Body Cycle

The third body cycle is the assimilation cycle and is from 8pm to 4am. This is the time the food you have eaten during the day is assimilated, absorbed and distributed throughout your body through your blood. It is the time where digested food moves into the colon as chime and is stored there for elimination. And, you should be eliminating this chime or fecal matter, when you wake up or during the morning, up to 12 noon.

Food that was eaten during the second

cycle, 12 noon to 8 p.m. and that was combined and eaten properly will digest within 3 to 4 hours. Whereas, food not combined properly, a meal consisting of protein, carbohydrates, soda, and other food will take up to 4 to 6 hours to pass through the stomach. During this time, some of your food will putrefy and ferment and become acidic. Under these conditions, you will not get many nutrients from that meal.

So, eat your last meal by 6-7pm, so that your food digests in your stomach by the time you go to bed. After three hours, your food will have moved into your small intestine where it is ready for assimilation.

When you go to bed 3 hours after your last meal, the next 6 hours, until 4am, your body will be absorbing the food you have eaten the previous day and moving waste into your colon and kidney.

Remember, anything you do different

than what these cycles call for will disrupt them and cause them to become extended. When this happens, your food turns into acid, you don't absorb the value of your food, you lose energy and become tired, and over time you gain weight and create constipation and other serious illnesses.

Just start changing your eating habits slowly, and as time passes, you will be doing more and more of what your body's natural cycles need.

9: How Acid Reflux Is Affected By An Acid Body

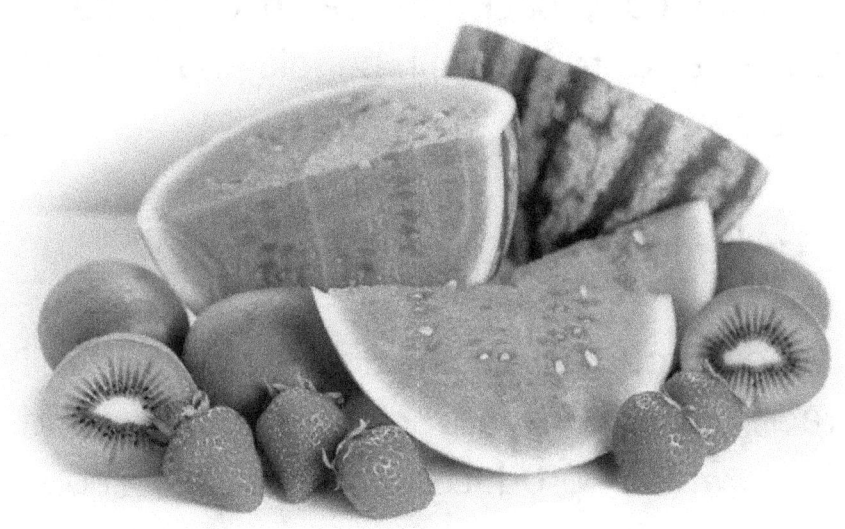

Minerals

Moving your body more toward alkalinity is what will help you gain better health. If you have acid reflux, your whole body is out of balance, and your organs are working overtime to compensate for this out of balance condition. It is the minerals that strengthen your muscles and bones. They are necessary for the contraction and function of muscles and tissue.

In this chapter, you will discover how to bring your body back into balance. Once in balance, acid reflux will be eliminated and will be more difficult to create.

Acid-Alkaline Body

When you have an acid body, it will attract disease. It attracts pathogens, and water, which produces a diseased body associated with being overweight and lacking the proper nutrition.

An alkaline body prevents your body from becoming ill and forming deadly diseases, like stomach problems, joint problems, organ degradation, body pain, heart disease, or even cancer. If you are already sick, then all of the chemicals inside fruits will help to revive you to better health. This is provided that your tissue damage has not gone beyond repair.

The minerals most important in changing and maintaining your body in an alkaline condition are sodium, potassium, chloride, calcium, phosphorus, magnesium, and sulphur.

Now, how your body can become alkaline might become a little confusing at first because of the terms used.

Acid Binding

There are certain minerals that are called acid binding. And, these are minerals we said are the most important ones in fruits - Sodium, potassium, calcium, phosphorus, and magnesium - because they are acid binding.

What acid binding means is when you eat fruits with these minerals and various chemicals, the fruit chemicals react in your cells to create energy. This reaction in your cells produces an alkaline residue. It is this residue that combines with acids in your body and neutralizes them. These neutralized acids will be then be eliminated from your body through lungs, kidney, and colon.

If not all the acid toxins are captured by acid binding matter, the remaining acids can be neutralized by body stores of alkaline minerals. If you don't have a good store of alkaline minerals, then these acids will remain in your body weaken it and creating disease. But if you do have a good store of alkaline minerals, these minerals will find acids, capture them, and bind with them. Then these acids will be moved out of your body, by your urine, stools, and breath.

Having a strong esophagus, stomach, small intestine and colon are the key to fighting acid reflux.

So you can see the importance of getting a lot of alkaline minerals into your body. Without them, acids would not get eliminate from your body, and they would remain in your body tissue and continue their body damage. Acid binding minerals mainly come from eating vegetables and fruits.

Alkaline Binding

Now, there are also minerals that become **alkaline binding** instead of **acid binding** and these minerals are sulphur, chlorine, iodine, phosphorus, bromine, fluorine, copper, and silicon. It is these minerals that when digested by a cell will produce a salt that will bind with alkaline minerals. These trapped alkaline binding salts will be excreted through your urine and other elimination channels.

When alkaline minerals are trapped by an acid salt, the alkaline minerals are removed from your body and your body becomes more acidic. This is the condition you are trying to avoid.

Foods that are alkaline binding and remove the minerals that you need to make your body alkaline are meat, carbohydrates, some vegetables and some fruits.

Although you need to eat both foods that are acid binding or alkaline binding, you want to eat more of the acid binding foods. This will keep your body slightly alkaline.

Where do Acid Toxins Come From?

So why is the body overloaded with acid toxins? Why can't the liver take care of all these toxins? Your liver has the function to remove acid wastes from natural food that is created by food digestion and cell metabolism. When your body encounters acid wastes, such as food enhancers, dyes, preservatives, pesticides, and the variety of food additives, the liver does not always know how to break them down or make them harmless.

Acid waste can also be created in your stomach. These are residues from incomplete digestion. As this waste, passes into your small intestine, they can be absorbed, if your intestinal walls suffer from leaky gut syndrome, a condition where large molecules are allow to pass through the intestine wall. This acid waste then flows into the liver.

When your liver can't neutralize all acid waste, it instructs calcium to bind with these toxic acids and to take them far away from the blood stream.

Stress Creates Acids

Now, we have talked about acid toxins in the body that are brought in through food and the environment. But, there is another factor that creates acids in the body.

This other factor is emotions that are activated through life stresses, like work pressures, divorce, friendship problems, martial issues, and other similar situations.

These emotional problems create acidic molecules that embed themselves into your tissues just like food acids. These, again, can be removed with acid binding minerals.

Body Organs

All body organs, including your stomach, function to rid the body of acid waste or toxins. Lack of acid binding food causes the deterioration of these organs. Each organ has a specific function in the elimination and neutralization of acid wastes and it does this in conjunction with acid binding minerals.

Acid Binding Foods

Here is a list of the fruits that have the highest alkaline minerals and that you should be eating to eliminate your body acids.

The percentage assigned to these fruits is based on fresh fruits that are organic, not cooked, canned or mixed with sugar. If they are cook or otherwise processed in some fashion, this will reduce their effectiveness as an acid binding fruit. However, they will still be somewhat effective in acid binding.

Here is the list of fruits to eat and drink in the order of priority. These are the fruits to eat during cycle 1, morning breakfast.

1.   Fruits at 100% Acid Binding – Best fruits To Eat and Drink
Lemons, melons – any type, watermelon

2.   Fruits at 93% Acid Binding – Great fruits To Eat and Drink
Cantaloupes, dried dates, dried figs, limes, mango, papaya

3. Fruits at 87% Acid Binding – Still Great Fruits to Eat and Drink
Kiwis, passion fruit, pineapples, raisins, umeboshi plums

4. Fruits at 80% Acid Binding – Eat and Drink These Fruits
Apricots, avocados, bananas, fresh dates, fresh figs, currants, gooseberries grapes, grapefruits guavas, kumquats, nectarines, pears, persimmons, quince

5. Fruits at 73% Acid Binding – Still Good Fruits to Eat and Drink
Apples, organs, peaches, pomegranate, raspberries, sour grapes, strawberries

6. Fruits at 67% Acid Binding – Still Neutralizes Acids, Eat and Drink This fruit
Cherries

Fruits to Concentrate On

These are the fruits you should concentrate on eating. Also eat them every day, if possible, fresh lemon juice in the morning and watermelon during the day.

You can see which fruits give you the best acid binding effects. Eat these fruits every morning, and you will be taking a big step in reducing your acid reflux.

Vegetables that Bind Acids

Here is the list of vegetables to eat in order of priority. All of these vegetables will neutralize acid, since they contain minerals that are acid binding.

1. **Vegetables at 93% Acid Binding** – best vegetables to eat
   Kelp, Seaweed, Watercress, Asparagus

2. **Vegetables at 80% Acid Binding** – still the best to eat
   Lettuce Leaf, Oyster plant, Pumpkin,

Spinach, Squash, Peas, Carrots, Celery, Chard, Swiss, Dandelion greens

3. **Vegetables at 73% Acid Binding –** great vegetables to eat
Bamboo shoots, Beets, Broccoli, Cabbage, Cauliflower, Collards, Corn, sweet, Ginger (fresh), Mushrooms, Mustard greens, Onions, Pepper, Potatoes, Green, Lima, String, Potatoes

4. **Vegetables at 67% Acid Binding –** eat plenty of these
Brussel sprouts, Cucumbers, Eggplants, Okra, Onions, Radishes, Tomatoes

5. **Vegetable juices at 80% to 93% Acid Binding**
Parsley, wheat grass, carrot, celery, etc.

6. **Soy Bean Products at 60% Acid Binding –** limit your use of tofu since it is a genetically modified organism, GMO

Dried beans, Soy cheese, Soy milk, Tempeh, Tofu

Misc. Acid Binding Food

7. Starches at 80% Acid Binding

  Arrowroot flour

8. Sugar at 73% acid Binding
Honey

9. Nuts and Seeds at 60 % to 67% Acid Binding
Almonds, sesame seeds, Granola, Essene Bread, Chestnuts

10. Misc. foods at 60% Acid Binding
Horseradish, Amaranth, Millet, Quinoa, Dried beans, Soy cheese, Soy milk,

NOTE: The lower the alkaline binding percentage, the more the food produces acid in your body.

11. All oils are basically at 50% and are considered neutral.
This includes almond, avocado, canola, coconut, corn castor, olive, soy, sunflower oil.

12. Beans, starches, and nuts and seeds are at 40% to 46% Alkaline Binding

Aduki, Black, Broadbean, Garbanzo, Mung, Pinto, Barley, Corn Meal, Lentils, Brans, Cashews, Coconut (dried), Pecans, Brans, Millet, Filberts, Walnuts, Pumpkin, Sunflower

13. Starches are at 26 to 33 % Alkaline Binding

Brown Rice, Buckwheat, Oats, Spelt, Wheat Whole, Peanuts, corn, rye

14. Rice at 20% Alkaline Binding

White rice

15. Sugar at 13% Alkaline Binding

White beet or cane sugar

Meat and Fish that Are Alkaline binding

16. Meat at 26% alkaline binding

Fish With fins and scales, Shellfish - shrimp, scallops, crab lobster, oyster

17. Meat at 20% Alkaline Binding

Chicken, turkey, rabbit

18. Meat at 13% Alkaline Binding

Beef, goat, pork, lamb

19. All oils are basically at 50% and are considered neutral.

This includes almond, avocado, canola, coconut, corn castor, olive, soy, sunflower oil.

20. Misc. Products at 13% to 26% Alkaline Binding

Liquor, wine, beer, coffee, black tea, caffeine drinks

You should be eating 80% acid binding foods and 20% alkaline binding foods. When you eat with this 80/20 formula, you will have an alkaline body over a period of time. Just gradually work toward this formula.

These are the basic eating principle you should use to achieve ultimate health.

10: Digestive Enzymes, Probiotics For Acid Reflux

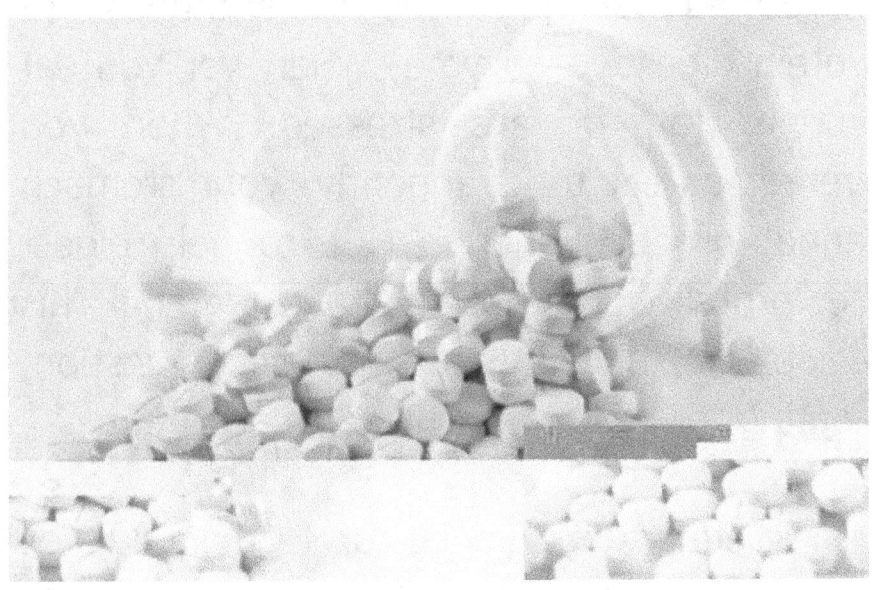

Digestion and Assimilation

Improving your digestion and assimilation of the foods you are eating are critical for getting rid your acid reflux.

Digestion and assimilation of food starts in your mouth. As your food travels into your stomach, Hydrochloric Acid, HCL, works on the protein and in your small intestine digestive enzymes complete the breakdown of your food.

Your stomach produces HCL and pepsin (a protein digestive enzyme) whenever you eat protein, fat, or are stressed. When you overeat or eat too frequently, your stomach cannot produce enough HCL to help digest the protein or fat you have eaten. This results in incomplete protein digestion, bloating, or gas and can lead to acid reflux.

Secreting good levels of HCL stimulates pepsin production and activates the pancreas to release adequate levels of digestive enzymes. The enzymes from the pancreas continue digestion of protein, fats and carbohydrates in the small intestine.

Digestive Enzymes

Eating a healthy diet, less food or protein at a sitting, and reducing stress can help return your HCL levels back to normal.

Anyone with digestive problems should take digestive enzyme supplements. The older you get the more important it is to take this supplement. As you age, secretions from various organs start to diminish and your body is deprived of these needed secretions.

Take digestive enzymes 30-45 minutes before meals to improve your digestion. If you forget to take enzymes before eating take them while eating or after. Taking digestive enzymes between meals can help with food allergies.

If you suffer from acid reflux, it is important to take digestive enzymes to help you digest your food. If you have developed stomach or small intestine ulcers, then you need to avoid using digestive enzymes.

In, Staying Healthy with Nutrition, 1992, Elson M. Hass, M.D. says,

"I have come to believe the digestive tract

and its function may be the single most important body component determining health and disease. Maintaining normal digestion, assimilation, and elimination is a necessity, and when these functions are faulty, we may not be aware these dysfunctions are contributing to so many other problems...Thus, when they are needed supplemental support of digestive enzymes may be even more important than HCL."

HCL supplements can be obtained as betaine hydrochloride. It can be found as a single supplement or in combination with other digestive enzymes.

Bromelain

Bromelain helps to digest protein. It also thins blood, so it is best not to take it when using the blood thinning drugs Coumadin and Warfarin. If you get any allergic reactions to Bromelain, stop using it right away.

Bromelain also has the ability to increase the effectiveness of any antibiotics you take.

Bromelain is found in pineapples and is useful in digesting protein. It has other benefits, such as reducing inflammation and platelet aggregation and clot formation. Bromelain is useful when there is a decrease in the enzymes produced by the pancreas.

There are some people that are allergic to pineapples, so they should not take Bromelain. As a digestive aid, use Bromelain with meals. As an anti- inflammation nutrient, use it between meals.

Recommended Bromelain dose is 1400 – 1800 MCU each day. If you are pregnant, it is considered safe to use Bromelain. Always try to use pineapples in your smoothies.

Papain

Papain, a mild digestive enzyme, is found

in papayas and helps in protein digestion. Use them as lozenges or as pills. Use papayas in your smoothies, when possible.

Amylase, Proteases and Lipases

Amylases, proteases, and lipases are the major group of digestive enzymes, which are secreted by the pancreas. Amylase digests carbohydrates, protease digest protein, and lipase digests fats. These enzymes are available in capsules and should be taken just before you eat.

It is best to use enteric enzymes, which are capable of reaching the small intestine, where they are needed. These enzymes are coated so they can pass through your stomach HCL without getting used up. As you age, your production of these enzymes decreases, so it is important to always take a digestive supplement.

Peppermint Capsules

Using enteric peppermint capsules can lower the pressure in your stomach, reducing the potential for reflux. A side benefit of this capsule is elimination of H. pyloric, the stomach bacteria that cause peptic ulcers.

Use these capsules 3 to 4 weeks at 200 mg/capsule, between meals, three times a day

Good Bacteria

If you are taking antibiotics, for sure, you need to take a "good bacteria" supplement. Antibiotics will kill both bad and good bacteria in your stomach and colon, allowing the bad bacteria to become more dominant. When this happens, you are more susceptible to creating an unbalance throughout your gastro-intestinal tract, which will affect the health of your entire body.

Acidophilus is a good bacteria. It must be the dominant bacteria in your colon; otherwise, you will be susceptible to many colon problems, including constipation.

How can you bring good bacteria like acidophilus into your colon? The stomach acids and the high alkaline environment of the small intestine prevent any reasonable amount of acidophilus to reach your colon. And, any acidophilus that does reach your colon will most likely be attacked and destroyed by the bad bacteria. If your colon is toxic and alkaline, this furthers the chances that acidophilus will be destroyed in your colon.

It is best to first feed your good bacteria with milk whey so that they become healthy, strong and can multiple. Once this is done, you can reestablish a high-level of good bacteria in your colon. Now, you can take acidophilus and other good bacteria capsules.

Take 2-3 **regular** capsules of good bacteria between meals with distilled water so to not activate the high levels of destructive stomach acid.

Taking 2-3 **enteric** capsules of good bacteria so the good bacteria by passes your stomach acids and reaches the small intestine.

Feeding the good bacteria milk whey

One of the best ways to increase the good bacteria in your colon is to feed the existing good bacteria so they become healthy. Taking 3 - 4 tablespoons in 8 oz. of water of edible-grade dairy whey does this. This should be done daily for 3 – 8 weeks.

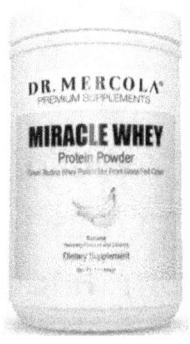

Web Link for Edible Whey

You can order this product at Amazon.com Add whey to your morning cereal, smoothies, or distilled water. **FructoOligosaccharides (FOS)**

If you cannot digest milk, then you can feed the good bacteria with FOS, a short-chain polysaccharides, which is a carbohydrate found in some grains, fruits and herbs. This carbohydrate is a natural complex of sugar. Since FOS is only partially digested in the intestines, it reaches your colon where it is the food used by good bacteria. Providing food to good bacteria helps to strengthen, stabilize, and multiple them in your colon. FOS also helps to clean your colon and build the cells in your colon wall.

Other carbohydrates that reach your colon undigested are called GOS, Galactooligosaccharides and inulin.

Providing FOS, GOS, and inulin supplements to your diet will increase absorption of calcium and magnesium and help to remove toxic material from your colon.

Some foods that contain FOS are Jerusalem artichokes, onions, leeks, burdock, chicory, garlic, and asparagus.

Because FOS is not available in the many foods you eat, it may be necessary for you to take it as supplement, while you are working on rebuilding your colon function.

The FOS recommended dose for promoting good bacteria in your colon is 3000 mg each day, taken during meals.

11: Herbs That Relieve Acid Reflux

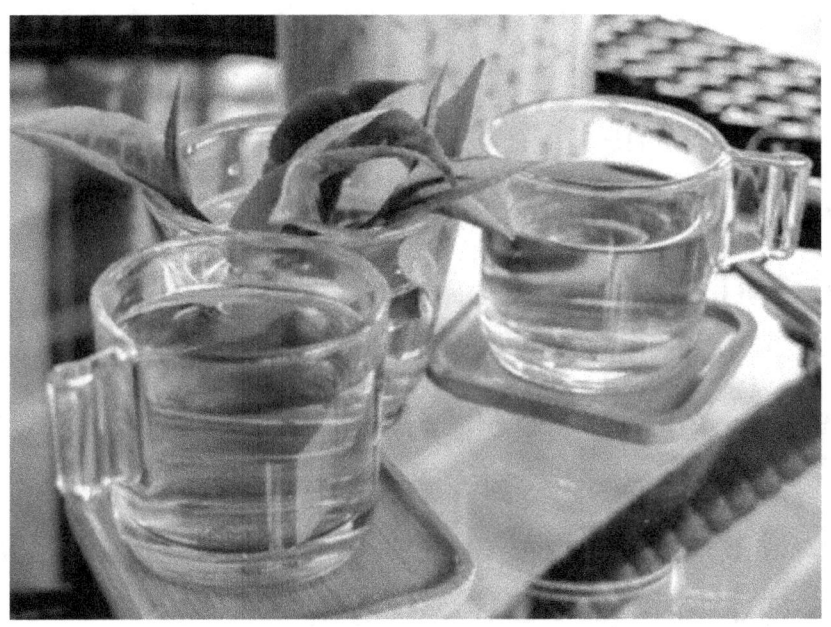

Cinnamon

Cinnamon has many medicinal uses aside from being great for various pastries. It has an antiseptic effect and has been historically used for colds and flu's. It has fighting power against Candida albicans and has the ability to settle acidic stomachs.

Here's how to use cinnamon for an acid stomach or heartburn:

- Toast raisin bread
- Butter the raisin bread, do not use margarine
- Sprinkle cinnamon on the bread
- Sprinkle cardamom on the bread

When you eat this toasted bread, chew slowly and completely, before swallowing to allow the digestive juices in your mouth to start breaking down this food.

Cardamom, which is found in India, has been used successful in treating Celiac disease, which is intolerance to gluten found in most bread.

Grapefruit Skins

Here is a way to settle your acid reflux

stomach with grapefruit. Use only organic grapefruit for this remedy.

Here's what to do:

- Grate the entire outer skin of an organic grapefruit
- Spread them out on a flat dish to dry
- Allow them to get crinkly dry
- Store them in a glass jar or zip lock bag

Whenever, you get an upset stomach, acid reflux or heartburn, start chewing and eating these strips of dried grapefruit. These strips will settle your stomach. Eat only a few of them and test to see how many you need.

Mace, Nutmeg, and Slippery Elm

Here is a natural remedy that uses mace and nutmeg, which has a history of treating indigestion, acid stomach, heartburn, acid reflux, stomach gas, and vomiting.

Here's how to use it with half and half dairy product and slippery elm root herb. Slippery elm herb can be purchase in any herb store in powder.

- 1 teaspoon of slippery elm bark
- a pinch of nutmeg
- a pinch of mace
- add distilled water to make a smooth slurry
- heat a pint of half and half to boil
- pull half and half from stove and add herb slurry
- stir in herb slurry

Allow this mixture to cool. Drink up to ½ cup at a time. Store the unused portion in the refrigerator. When drinking the next cup, warm this mixture up.

Acid reflux and heartburn require alkaline nutrients to provide relief. These 4 natural remedies, when prepared properly, will give you the relief you need from these conditions. Try them; you will be surprised on how well they work.

More Remedies

Here is a list of natural remedies that you can use when you have acid reflux or heartburn. No need to use antacids, which have unwanted side effects and contain aluminum.

Anise and peppermint

Here's a tea that you can make to help you with acid reflux or heartburn. It will help you reduce the amount of acid you have in your stomach. Mix together equal amounts of aniseed, peppermint and lavender. Make an infusion of this tea:

- boiling 2 ½ cup distilled water
- pour this water over a teaspoon or more of the herbal mixture
- let this tea sit for 3- 5 minutes
- strain the tea and add a little bit of honey, if you like place this tea in a thermos
- Drink up to 8 oz. in the morning and 8 oz. in the evening to get relief of acid reflux.

Aniseed or anise – is a powerful herb that helps in digestive conditions and has many other benefits for your body. Use only the ash-colored anise called green anise, European anise or sweet anise. There are two other types of anise, star anise and caraway, which should not be used here.

Peppermint – is another powerful herb for stomach conditions or heartburn. It helps in digestion, stomach distension, cramps, ulcers, and gas. Use it in tea form.

Betaine, Pepsin, and Papaya digestive enzymes

As you get older, your stomach weakens in its ability to produce hydrochloric acid to digest protein. It is undigested protein that leads to acid reflux or heartburn. Use digestive enzymes that contain Betaine, pepsin, or HCl with each meal to make sure you digest all of your protein.

Papaya digestive enzymes, which contain papain, are also excellent for protein digestion, and you can use them with each meal. Use 500mg or more of papaya enzymes per meal.

Pineapples

Pineapples are a store house of enzymes and contain bromelain, an enzyme that reduces protein. Pineapples support digestion, reduce inflammation, and supports wound healing. The fresh juice has a high level of enzymes that will help you stop your acid reflux. You can also buy bromelain as tablet and take 200 – 500mg per meal.

Ginger Tea

Drink ginger tea around 30 minutes before bedtime. This will help you reduce the risk of acid reflux.

Chamomile Tea

You can drink chamomile tea to relax. Stress is one of the factors that can lead to reflux.

Mustard

To relieve heartburn, take a teaspoon of mustard.

12: A Super Herb For Acid Reflux

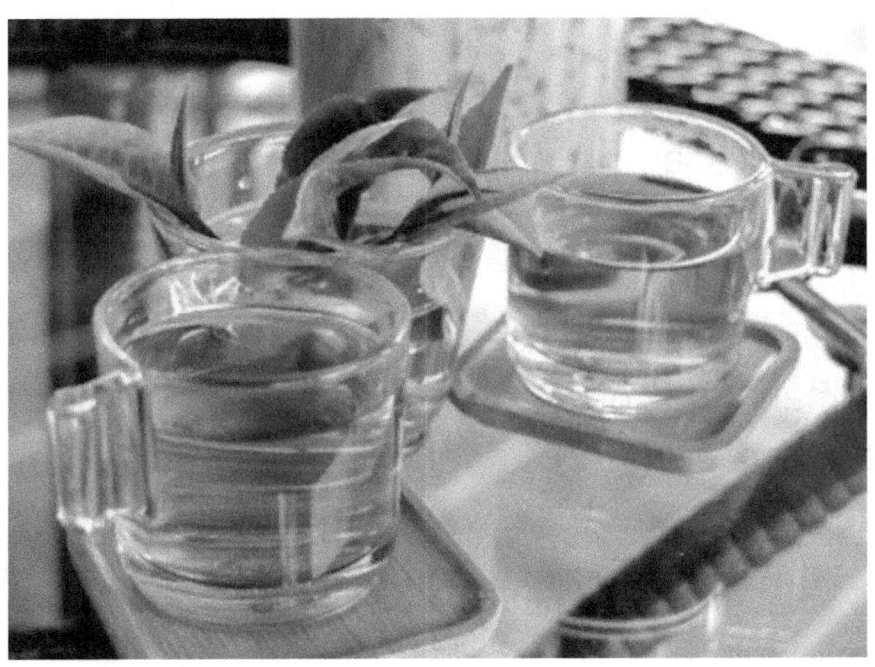

Licorice

In the 1940's, licorice was discovered to be useful in treating peptic ulcers. Unfortunately, it had side effects that lead to high blood pressure, potassium loss, and fluid retention.

Researchers discovered that the ingredient in licorice that caused those side effects was "glycyrrhizin." They were able to remove 97% of this chemical and the result was a product call "deglycyrrhizinated" licorice, DGL. DGL had the same healing properties as plain licorice and had no side effects.

DGL was first used to heal ulcers in the stomach and duodenum without suppressing stomach acids. DGL worked just as good as the drug Zantac or Tagamet that are designed to suppress stomach acid.

As more people used DGL, they found they got relief from a variety of stomach issues – heartburn, acid reflux, indigestion, bloating, and gas. In addition, they found using DGL was better than using antacids or acid blockers.

DGL works by improving and restoring the integrity of the esophageal, stomach and duodenum lining. It does this by promoting mucus release and cell rebuilding. The mucus released provides gastrointestinal lining protection from acids and gives the lining time to rebuild and regenerated. The result is healing and strengthening of the affected tissue.

Here's how to use DGL. DGL comes in large tablets that you place in your mouth to melt. You can chew them slightly, but do not swallow them, since it is your salvia that helps activate the DGL.

By allowing DGL to melt in your mouth, the resulting liquid will now run along your esophagus and start the healing process, where ever there is tissue inflammation or damage.

Use two tablets 3-4 times a day on an empty stomach. Do not use any water, when you are taking the tablets. You can take the tablets at least an hour before you eat or an hour after.

Although DGL provides relief for heartburn, acid reflux and other stomach disturbances, it does not totally provide a cure. It does provide recover from damaged gastrointestinal lining as occurs with ulcers, but does not change the level of stomach acid. For a cure, use DGL and the eating and lifestyle recommendations provided in this book.

In most all cases, acid reflux is caused by too little or too much stomach acid. When too little acid is causing acid reflux, it makes no sense to use antacids or acid blocking drugs, which decrease your stomach acid even more. Low levels of stomach acid usually lead to serious illnesses.

Because so much is still unknown about the actual causes of acid reflux, it is known that DGL can give you some acid reflux relief and in some mild cases cure it.

Use DGL for mild or severe cases of acid reflux and you will be surprised at the results you get.

13: Strengthening Your Lower Esophageal Sphincter

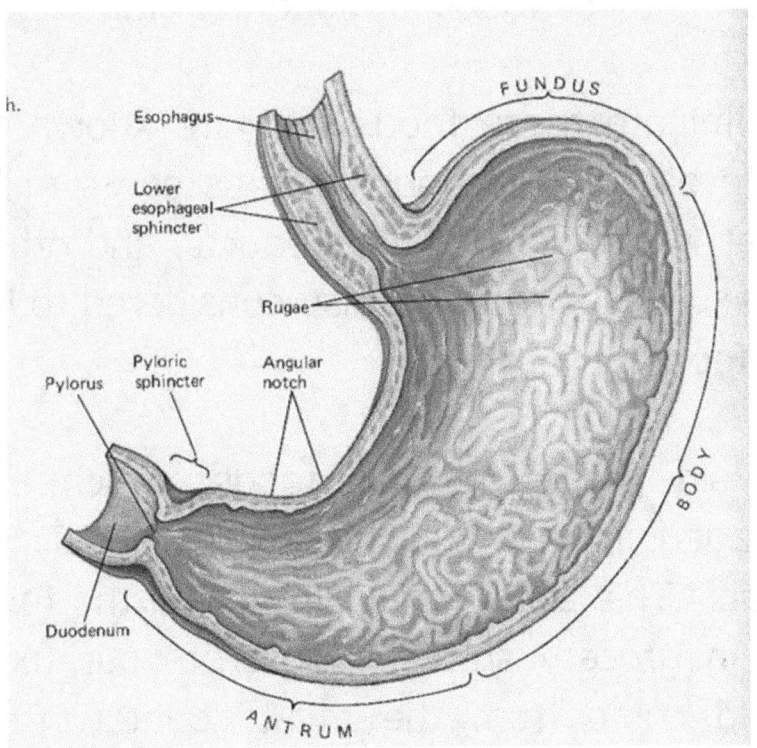

Strengthening the LES

Here are some natural steps that you can use to strengthen your Lower Esophageal

Sphincter valve:

First, these foods can weaken the LES valve – coffee, peppermint, spearmint, sugar, chocolate, onions, and alcohol. Once you have strengthened your LES, you can return to eating these foods in moderate amounts.

Eliminate those foods that are known to create allergic reactions such as cow's milk, wheat, white flour, diary products, and other foods. These foods are also considered to be acid foods.

Avoid processed acid foods, which are packaged in cans, bags, cartons, paper, or plastic. This covers pretty much all the food sold in grocery stores. Most of your food should come from the meat counter, fruit and vegetable area, seed bins, nut bins, oat and bran bins, and natural grains section. You should also be going to your farmers market each week.

Avoid overeating and having a large amount of food in your stomach. Excess food in your stomach can increase your stomach gas pressure and force your LES valve to weaken or open. Give your LES valve time to gain strength by not exposing it to excessive stomach pressure.

Avoid using certain drugs, although this might be impossible. If you take drugs, perhaps you can start looking for and start using some natural remedies, so that you can lessen the use of drugs.

Here are some of the drugs at cause LES problems – NSAID's, bronchodilators, channel blockers, beta-blockers, antianxiety drugs, and nitroglycerine. These drugs relax the muscles around the LES valve causing them to open during normal stomach gas pressures.

Watch how you do certain physical activities, such as waist bending, staining during bowel movements, coughing, and lifting heavy objects. This increases the pressure in the stomach, causing the LES valve to open.

After a meal do not lie down. This causes food to flow back towards the LES valve putting pressure on it. So it is a good idea to eat your last meal around two to three hours before bedtime.

There you have it, some natural remedies and activities that strengthen or weaken your LES valve. Just applying some or all these will result in reducing the frequency of your acid reflux and heartburn.

If you have acid reflux or heartburn, using natural remedies to rebalance your stomach is what nature intended. In the next chapter, you will find more ideas to help with your acid reflux.

14: How to Fix Your Acid Reflux

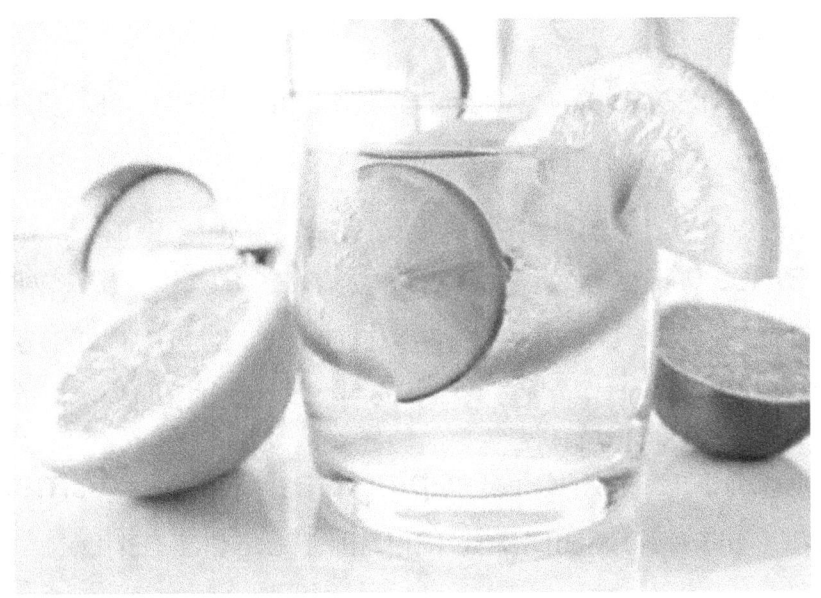

Acid Reflux can be Serious

Acid reflux is not a serious condition if it happens infrequently, but can be uncomfortable. If you are experiencing reflux weekly, then you need to pay attention and take this problem serious. Frequent acid reflux bouts can turn in an esophagus ulcer or cancer.

Reflux that occurs weekly is considered GERD or a disease. You can consult your doctor to get help. And, by using many of the lifestyle, dietary, and natural remedy changes, you can overcome and eliminate reflux for good.

At heart of the reflux problem is how, when, and what you eat. Your stomach functions in a specific way and if you go against this way, you will end up with indigestion, bloating, heartburn, stomach pain, diarrhea, vomiting, and weight gain.

Concentrating keeping a good stomach function can help you eliminate acid reflux.

Fixing Your Acid Reflux

Use these steps in dealing with your acid reflux or GERD. You don't have to apply all of these immediately. Just start doing one or two per day. Do a major change one a week.

Step one

Review chapter 4 and eliminate some of

the conditions that contribute to acid reflux. This includes physical things you can do and the foods to avoid. And, review the saliva test and start testing.

Step two

Review your lifestyle and make some changes in how and what you eat.

Include more fiber into your diet by eating high fiber foods.

Step Three

See what changes you can make to get into alignment with your three body cycles.

Step Four

Start eating those foods that will make your body more alkaline.

Step Five

Use digestive enzymes, probiotics, and natural remedies to get natural relief for your acid reflux.

Step Six

Start some activity that will help you strengthen your LES.

Final Thoughts

Most people have digestive problems that create a variety of illness as they age. These illnesses are not a result of aging, but a result of the food they eat or over eat. As has already been said many times, we eat more junk, processed, and packaged food than our stomach can digest. We eat more meat and protein then we should. We drink more unusual drinks that are mainly sugar.

We need to eat more live vegetables and fruits. This will minimize any acid reflux problems you might have and keep your body alkaline. If you have poor health then you have an acid body. When you mentally decided to make your body alkaline, it may take 3 to 12 months to see some results.

And, this may depend on how acidic your body is.

Your body is designed to be electrically balanced. This is done by eating both acid and alkaline foods. If you eat too much of an acid food or alkaline food, you move towards illness. Acid reflux is one of these illnesses.

When too much acid food is eaten, your stomach can't completely digest it. The excess undigested food turns into an acid waste that needs to be removed from the body. This waste causes stomach spasms or twitching that causes an increase in stomach gas that pops open the valve between the esophagus and stomach.

Acidic stomach content is sucked into the esophagus causing a burning sensation in the chest and throat. This is acid reflux resulting in heartburn.

The nutritional suggestions given here will go a long way in getting you past your acid reflux. Slowly start adding many of these eating ideas presented here into your lifestyle. They are good not just for Acid reflux or heartburn, but they can serve as your foundation to gaining better health in all parts of your body.

15: About The Author And Other Resources

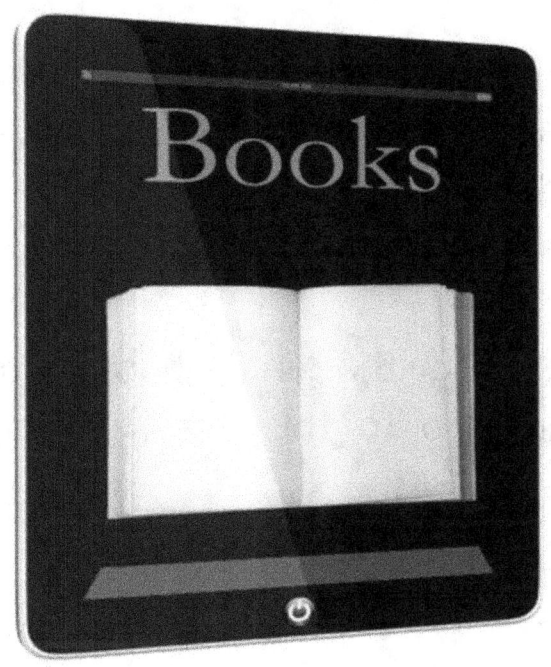

Rudy Silva is a natural consultant nutritionist educated in the United State in Nutrition and Physics. He is a graduate from the San Jose State University in California. He is author of 40 other e-books on natural remedies. He has authored a newsletter in natural remedies for over 4 years. He has websites promoting special recommended products and information.

Resource page

Here are some of the other kindle e-books about natural remedies that have been written by this author. You can see the entire list at:

To see all of the kindle books written by this author, go to this the Authors Profile Page or this URL:

http://tinyurl.com/b2f7wd3

If you need support or want to promote any of his e-books, please contact him at rss41@yahoo.com and expect a reply within 24 hours. He looks forward to hearing from you and is happy to help you understand his material on natural and nutritional health.

Give a Review

And, don't forget to give a review for this e-book at Amazon so that others can gain the benefits of what is in this e-book.

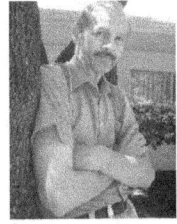

To you, for creating better health and more happiness in your life,

Rudy S Silva

www.ingramcontent.com/pod-product-compliance
Lightning Source LLC
Chambersburg PA
CBHW072248310526
45795CB00011B/354